14 NEW WAYS TO

STOP

MASTURBATION

By Olutoke Akande

Contents

INTRODUCTION

Masturbation has become an issue all over the world, there is no race or tribe that doesn't masturbate, and even among the major religion like Christian, Muslims, many of their followers or people are involving in masturbation secretly. But most of the major religions are condemning the act.

At early stage most we young boys take this as an opportunity to test their joysticks, to know how active their machine can perform. It is a thing of pride at that early stage; most of them believe that whenever they masturbate and milk comes out from their joysticks that show that they have turned to men.

When I was age 14, I and my friend went to the bathroom to take our bath; suddenly my friend came up with this topic about masturbation. He told me that I am not yet a man, I reply why you are saying I am not yet a man. He said that my joystick has not started bringing out milk, I laugh and I told him that I masturbate yesterday and I saw a milk coming out from my joystick, Which he congratulate me and said you have become a man.

At that early stage we the young guys believe that slitting out milk from our joysticks makes us men, as at then, we normally brag about it all the time.

I will like you to pay attention to what I am going to teach concerning how you can stop masturbation without stress.

If you have become addicted to masturbation that means you are in trouble, because it is going to be difficult to let it go, but don't worry, because after you read and followed all the steps with all sincerity inside this book you are going to gain your freedom from the hand of this muster called masturbation.

Many books authors are saying that it is difficult to stop masturbation. But I am telling you with all authority that those books authors are lying. With my book, you are going to have your freedom from masturbation that has colonized your joystick for many years. You know how many years you have been masturbating if yours is five years that mean masturbation has colonized your joystick for the past five years.

Something about this masturbation is that, If you have turned it to hobbies or you are the type that excessively masturbates, you are going to find it difficult to have an interest in the opposite sex, if care is not taking you may end up without having a wife or get married.

Masturbation can completely destroy your life, I'm talking seriously. If you jerk off frequently, you can become addicted. And unfortunately, you may end up needing your daily dose of jerking off. I have a guy who masturbates so much that he put masturbation in his hobbies list. When my friend is bored, he will go to the bathroom take a shower, a little soap or oil and, bam, he's in heaven.

If you masturbate every day, you will allow this act as part of your daily life, along with eating food, going to work, to school, face book, and twitter with drinking water every day.

If you want to stop masturbation you have to follow all the steps that I am about to list below, if you want to stop masturbation within a week or less than a week you have to take those steps seriously. A lot of my readers have followed those steps and they have seen the result. You have to be sincere with yourself if you wanted to have a good result; those steps below have helped a lot of people I know, so you have to put all your best to achieve a fantastic result.

CHAPTER1. BY MARRIAGE

The first step toward how you can stop masturbation is to get married. Without that you will find it difficult to let your masturbation lover go, you have to replace it with your wife. You have to get rid of your old life style or else there will be no room for your new life style. So you have to sacrifice one for the others.

Frankly speaking, marriage has helped a lot of men and women to overcome frequent jerking off all the time. I have a friend he is the type of friend that jerk off frequently when he was still single back then in college, we were to together in the same department. I know more about him very well, he is my close guy. One day he told me that since when he got married to his beautiful queen he has no time to masturbate again because he always satisfies himself whenever he is making love with his wife. He told me that he hates masturbation because it irritates him whenever he wanted to try it .this is a guy that masturbate like a person that is drinking water, then in the college.

You can see marriage is an important tool to use, if you really wanted to stop masturbation for life, marriage has helped a lot of guys I know to overcome masturbator.

CHAPTER2. HAVE MORE THAN ONE GIRLFRIEND

I know, you guys will be thinking why I said you should have more than one girlfriend. Don't worry about that, I am going to explain the reason why I said you should have more than one girlfriend.

Seriously speaking having just one girlfriend

May not help at all, if you really wanted to stop masturbation, sometimes we know how selfish some girlfriend can be especially when they are not in good terms with you. They may not give you access to their subway; I mean sex. And you don't know how long she may starve you.

Even some married men are passing through this same problem at home, sometimes their wife can be selfish due to a reason is best known to them. If you are the type that whenever you and your wife are having some misunderstanding at home and she dined you of sex at night, I am sorry to say this you have to look for option B or else it may bring you back to masturbation that you have left for a long time.

If you wanted to keep a girlfriend you have to be careful so that you wife will not catch you in the act.

Because of the bad attitude of some women towards their husband, this has increased the numbers of men cheating on their wife. Because their wife use to dined them sex whenever they are not in good terms.

Since the introduction of sex toys, many men are saying that they cannot cope with their wife anymore, that they have tired of their wife nagging all the time at home, so they prefer having their sex toys around them should being a case they are in the mood.

So having just one girlfriend around is bad you have to have more girlfriends should being the case you and the other one are not in good terms, you can satisfy your self with the other girlfriends this will help you to stop masturbating.

CHAPTER3. STOP WASHING PORNOGRAPHY

If you know that you don't have a girlfriend or wife, I will advise you to stop washing porn. Because it will force you to masturbate. Porn is meant for those married people or for those that have a girlfriend, they use this porn to kick start their mood whenever they wanted to have sex with their partners.

Married couple also uses porn to learn styles that are trending. For guys that are still single and you know that you don't have a girlfriend, you have to stop washing porn from your laptop computer or from your phone. You have to delete them from your laptop and phone if you really wanted to stop masturbation. I don't see the reason why you are saying that you wanted to stop masturbating; still, you keep on downloading latest and old schools porn on your phones and laptops from the internet. That shows that you are not ready to stop the bad habit yet.

There are a lot of things to let go if you really wanted to stop masturbation, though it is not that easy, you have to remain committed and focus. You have to set a target that by this time next week you will be free from it.

You have to avoid those romance movies especially if you know that you are still single without a girlfriend, stay away from movies like Game of the throne, Spartacus, the Rome. Those movies may put you in the mood to masturbate.

CHAPTER4. KEEP YOURSELF BUSY WITH OTHER THINGS

Keeping yourself busy can really go a long way if you are ready to stop masturbation. You can think of any new things to learn during your idle time, or staying at home doing nothing. Research has proven that most of those guys involving in masturbation are the idle one, they always stay at home doing nothing.

Try to engage yourself, by doing or learn something new this will make you forget about masturbation. Sublimate by doing things like drawing, learning how to play a musical instrument, writing, you can also involve in games like soccer, table tennis, swimming, horse riding e.t.c. you can also enroll in a driving school where you are going to learn how to drive cars. If you love cooking you can also enroll yourself in any cooking school, involving yourself with different kind of activities will make you forget about masturbation.

CHAPTER5. PATRONIZE THE PROSTITUTE

I know some of the guys out there will like to sentence me to 21 years in prison for saying this. But don't worry I am going to explain it in the way you are going to agree with me. The reason why I make use of this point is that we have some guys out there that are very shy to talk to a girl, they cannot even express their feeling to any girl that they love to go out with or have has a girlfriend.

Most of those shy guys believe that since they cannot talk to a girl due to their condition they rather masturbate. Remember masturbation is a bad habit that you need to let go.

Going to the prostitute is never bad ideas to do, a prostitute is a human bean they are not mustered, but you have to protect yourself with condom whenever you are having fun with them. Don't use your naked joystick on their subway just like that, always remember to use a condom.

Even the so called married men are patronizing those prostitutes because their wife can be selfish sometimes. I am advising those shy guys out there instead of masturbation they should patronize the prostitute. during the withdrawal period from masturbation, especially if you're a world class champion in this category, you will feel a strong need and develop a strong appetite, two elements that will naturally help motivate you to talk to women and try to sleep with them.

As a shy guy the more you are patronizing the prostitute you are going to develop the confidence to associate yourself with girls, before you will realize it you have started expressing your feeling to other girls who are not even a prostitute with confident. This is just a gradual process it may take time before it will materialize. Going to the prostitute will help you to stop masturbation.

CHAPTER6. STAY AWAY FROM HARD DRUGS

The reason why you have to stay away from hard drugs is that it makes you do some nasty thing that you don't suppose to do. Hard drugs will make you do something stupid because you are not in your right senses. Like masturbating; total abstinence from drugs will make you think straight, it will open your mind towards the new thing and allowed you to focus your mind on new things. Staying away from drugs will make you stop masturbation. Remember that excessive masturbation is a symptom of another problem

CHAPTER7. YOGA AND ECKANKAR EXERCISE

Yoga exercise is one of the effective measures to cure the sensitivity of masturbation problems. As long as one practice yoga exercise the beneficial impact are going to be visible to that person. Eckankar exercise is another way to stop masturbation; this exercise will develop your spiritual life and open your mind towards important things of life. Just close your two eyes, breathe in and out with your nose three to five times then concentrate on your forehead then chant the lettered world HU for like 15-20 minute do this every day before going to bed, you notice that the habit of masturbation will no longer be their again in your life. This Eckankar exercise will make you worry less, no more love, feel energized; it will make you change your bad habit

CHAPTER8. STOP THINKING ABOUT SEX

If you are serious about quitting masturbation you must stop thinking about sex all the time. Try to focus your mind on other things that are more beneficial, something that you are going to benefit from in due time. Like reading your books, dancing, you can even volunteer yourself to help people around you.

Doing this will make your mind to stop thinking about sex all the time. Sometimes when we are lonely, we will be thinking about some crazy things in our mind. You may be thinking about a girl in your street that you saw last time before you will realize it, you will begin to imagine how you are going to have sex with her. By thinking this way you are going to develop that urge to masturbate, because you allowed the thought to run through your mind.

If you are serious about quitting masturbation you have to learn how to fixed your mind in other things apart from sex

CHAPTER9. HAVE MORE FRIENDS

Sometimes the reason behind your masturbation is because you always stay alone at home all the time that is why you always fall into the temptation to masturbate. If you have many friends, your friends may take you to a party to have some fun. Going out with your friend will make your mind not to think about masturbation again. Go out with your guys, always stay close with them and learn how to do the right thing

If you are the shy type it is good to go out with your friends to the clubs or to any birthday party, church programs or to any event around the town. This will keep you busy and your mind out of masturbation. If you find yourself masturbating out of loneliness, try to stay social. Join some social clubs, so you can be around people or join a dating site that you have someone on the internet to talk to. Soon you will learn how to avoid masturbation and will get into relationships instead. Try to stay out in public as much as possible so you won't be alone.

CHAPTER10. BUY A PET

Having a pet around can really help you to get rid of masturbation. When you have a pet at home, you have to concentrate your mind on taking care of your pet, doing this will keep you busy throughout the day. What is good about having a pet at home is that you will not be alone at home;   you and your pet will be playing together at home.

There are a lot of pet out there that you can buy with your money and also their food is very cheap also to buy. You can get up to two dogs or two cats it all depends on your choice, as for me I prefer having two at the same time. Sometimes it is very interesting washing the two of your pet playing together or fighting one another.

Sometimes that pet can make you see a thing in the other way round. You will be amazed how funny that pet can be, you can bring out you book and pen to write what you discover from your pet or if you have a video camera you can video them whenever they are doing something that is funny, Just post it in your website or blog, face book for your friends to wash or read, soon you will not have time to masturbate again.

CHAPTER11. WATCH OTHER INTERESTING TV SHOWS

One of the ways to get rid of masturbation is to look for any interesting TV show that you love to watch anytime that you are alone at home. If you know that you are not going out with your guys or hang out with them you can choose to watch something that interest you on the TV, there are a lot of TV shows all over the station that you can choose from. You can choose to watch reality shows, news, business news, politics, some sports game; you may even love to watch some movie series.

There are a lot of TV programs that you can watch on your TV, doing this will make you forget about masturbation. I like watching a soccer game, I can sit in front of my TV watching a football match from morning till night without going out, especially during the weekend.

I am a Manchester United fans, I love watching my team playing against another team during the weekend, doing this use to keep me busy through the day.

If you can also look for any interesting TV programs, you will find it amazing; you will no longer have time to masturbate anymore. By the time you keep your mind busy with other activities you are going to find it hard to masturbate.

CHAPTER12. LISTEN TO MUSIC

Music is part of our life; everybody loves to listen to music in one way or the other. It all depends on the types of music you love to listen to.

The reason why listening to music is very important is that music can change your mood. Whenever you are sad or you are passing through something, you can play your music to forget your sorrow and life will go on from there. The same thing also applies to when you are masturbating, if you wanted to stop masturbation you have to listen to music sometime when you are alone at home doing nothing so that you will not have the urge to masturbate.

CHAPTER13. GET RID OF SEX TOYS

If you are the type that use sex toys to jerk off all the time, this is the time to get rid of them, if you really wanted to stop masturbation. The more you keep them around the more you will be tempted to use them for self-servicing. So get all the toys together and destroy them, it is for your own good. When the urge is very intense take a cold shower instead.

CHAPTER14. STAY COMMITTED

You have to set a goal for yourself if you really wanted to stop masturbation. You need to set a target, that at the end of this week or month you are going to stop this shameful act, without that you are going to find it difficult to stop masturbation.

You have to stay focus when you are following all the steps that I listed in this book. The setting goal for yourself, start with going three days clean without masturbation. The third day is the speed bump, get past that and you know that you're committed. Then go a week, then 10-15 days, and then three weeks, and then 21 days, e.t.c. doing this have shown that you are committed to stopping masturbation before you will realize it you are going to notice that you don't masturbate anymore.

CONCLUSION

If you are serious about quitting masturbation you have to follow those steps that I listed in this book and be committed to it. Don't take any of the steps for granted, some of the steps may be difficult to practice but you just have to sacrifice your time and energy on them and put all your effort to it. If you wanted to get the best result you have to follow them and avoid some of the things that I said you should avoid for a better result.

Other Books by Olutoke Akande

1. Medicinal Honey and Healing Properties

2. Medicinal Honey

3. Easy Way to Stop Snoring Naturally

They are available in Amazon kindle book

www.ingramcontent.com/pod-product-compliance
Lightning Source LLC
Chambersburg PA
CBHW081258250726
48654CB00012B/1646